KETO DIET COOKBOOK

80 Healthy and Delicious Low-Carb recipes to Shed-Off Weight and Increase Your Energy Level

Written by

Sam Gallo

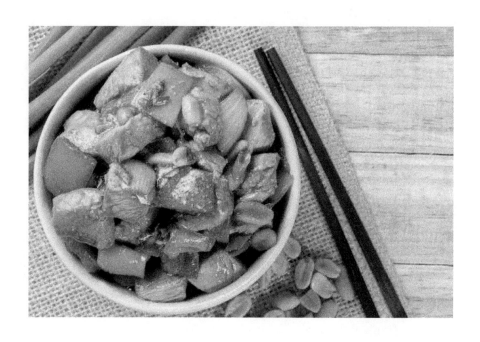

Table of Content

Introduction

Want to follow a ketogenic diet but not sure where to start? Struggling with finding delicious and tummy-filling recipes when going "against the grains"? Do not worry! In this book you will find mouth-watering delights for any occasion and any eater, you will not believe that these recipes will help you restore your health and slim down your body.

Successfully practiced for more than nine decades, the ketogenic diet hs proven to be the ultimate long-term diet for any person. The restriction list may frighten many, but the truth is, this diet is super adaptable, and the food combinations and tasty meals are pretty endless.

Most people believe that our bodies are designed to run on carbohydrates. We think that ingesting carbohydrates is the only way to provide our bodies with the energy they need to function normally. However, what many people don't know is that carbohydrates are not the only source of fuel our bodies can use. Our bodies can also use fat as an energy source! When we decide to ditch carbs and provide our bodies with more fat, then we've begun our journey into the ketogenic diet, and this cookbook will be the guide you need to make your journey simple and enjoyable...let's start!

Breakfast Recipes

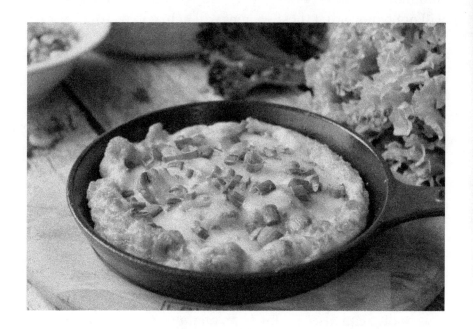

Vegetable & Blue Cheese Egg Scramble

Ingredients for 4 servings

1 tbsp butter

1 cup sliced white mushrooms

2 cloves garlic, minced

16 oz blue cheese

½ cup spinach, sliced

6 fresh eggs

Directions and Total Time: approx. 30 minutes

Melt butter in a skillet over medium heat and sauté mushrooms and garlic for 5 minutes. Crumble blue cheese into the skillet and cook for 6 minutes. Introduce the spinach and sauté for 5 more minutes. Crack the eggs into a bowl, whisk until well combined and creamy in color, and pour all over the spinach. Use a spatula to immediately stir the eggs while cooking, until scrambled and no more runny, about 5 minutes. Serve.

Per serving: Cal 469; Net Carbs 5g; Fat 39g; Protein 25g

Omelet Wrap with Avocado and Salmon

Ingredients for 2 servings

1 avocado, sliced

2 tbsp chopped chives

2 oz smoked salmon, sliced

1 spring onion, sliced

4 eggs, beaten

3 tbsp cream cheese

2 tbsp butter

Salt and black pepper to taste

Directions and Total Time: approx. 15 minutes

In a small bowl, combine the chives and cream cheese; set aside. Season the eggs with salt and pepper. Melt butter in a pan and add the eggs; cook for 3 minutes. Flip the omelet over and cook for another 2 minutes until golden. Remove to a plate and spread the chive mixture over. Top with salmon, avocado, and onion slices. Wrap and serve.

Per serving: Cal 514; Net Carbs 5.8g; Fat 47g; Protein 37g

Coconut Gruyere Biscuits

Ingredients for 4 servings

4 eggs

¼ cup butter melted

¼ tsp salt

1/3 cup coconut flour

¼ cup coconut flakes

½ tsp xanthan gum

¼ tsp baking powder

2 tsp garlic powder

¼ tsp onion powder

½ cup grated Gruyere cheese

Directions and Total Time: approx. 30 minutes

Preheat oven to 350 F. Line a baking sheet with parchment paper. In a food processor, mix eggs, butter, and salt until smooth. Add coconut flour, coconut flakes, xanthan gum, baking, garlic, and onion powders, and Gruyere cheese. Combine smoothly. Mold 12 balls out of the mixture and arrange on the baking sheet at 2-inch intervals. Bake for 25 minutes or until the biscuits are golden brown.

Per serving: Cal 267; Net Carbs 5.1g, Fat 26g, Protein 12g

Feta & Spinach Frittata with Tomatoes

Ingredients for 4 servings

5 oz spinach

8 oz feta cheese, crumbled

1 pint cherry tomatoes, halved

10 eggs

2 tbsp olive oil

4 scallions, diced

Directions and Total Time: approx. 35 minutes

Preheat oven to 350 F. Drizzle the oil in a casserole and place in the oven until heated. In a bowl, whisk eggs along with pepper and salt. Stir in spinach, feta cheese, and scallions. Pour the mixture into the casserole, top with the cherry tomatoes and place back in the oven. Bake for 25 minutes. Cut the frittata into wedges and serve with salad.

Per serving: Cal 461; Net Carbs 6g; Fat 35g; Protein 26g

Coconut Almond Muffins

Ingredients for 4 servings

2 cups almond flour

2 tsp baking powder

8 oz ricotta cheese, softened

¼ cup butter, melted

1 egg

1 cup coconut milk

Directions and Total Time: approx. 30 minutes

Preheat oven to 400 F. Grease a muffin tray with cooking spray. Mix flour, baking powder, and salt in a bowl.

In a separate bowl, beat ricotta cheese and butter using a hand mixer and whisk in the egg and coconut milk. Fold in almond flour and spoon the batter into the muffin cups two-thirds way up. Bake for 20 minutes, remove to a wire rack to cool slightly for 5 minutes before serving.

Per serving: Cal 320; Net Carbs 6g; Fat 30.6g; Protein 4g

Almond Butter Shake

Ingredients for 2 servings

3 cups almond milk

3 tbsp almond butter

⅛ tsp almond extract

1 tsp cinnamon

4 tbsp flax meal

1 scoop collagen peptides

A pinch of salt

15 drops stevia

Directions and Total Time: approx. 2 minutes

Add milk, butter, flax meal, almond extract, collagen, salt, and stevia to the blender. Blitz until uniform and smooth. Serve into smoothie glasses, sprinkled with cinnamon.

Per serving: Cal 326; Net Carbs 6g; Fat 27g; Protein 19g

Raspberry Mini Tarts

Ingredients for 4 servings

For the crust:

6 tbsp butter, melted

2 cups almond flour

1/3 cup xylitol

1 tsp cinnamon powder

For the filling:

3 cups raspberries, mashed

½ tsp fresh lemon juice

¼ cup butter, melted

½ tsp cinnamon powder

¼ cup xylitol sweetener

Directions and Total Time: approx. 25 min + chilling time

Preheat oven to 350 F. Lightly grease 4 mini tart tins with cooking spray. In a food processor, blend butter, almond flour, xylitol, and cinnamon. Divide the dough between the tart tins and bake for 15 minutes. In a bowl, mix raspberries, lemon juice, butter, cinnamon, and xylitol. Pour filling into the crust, gently tap on a flat surface to release air bubbles and refrigerate for 1 hour. Serve.

Per serving: Cal 435; Net Carbs 4.8g, Fat 29g, Protein 2g

Morning Beef Patties with Lemon

Ingredients for 6 servings

6 ground beef patties

4 tbsp olive oil

2 ripe avocados, pitted

2 tsp fresh lemon juice

6 fresh eggs

Red pepper flakes to garnish

Directions and Total Time: approx. 25 minutes

In a skillet, warm oil and fry patties for 8 minutes. Remove to a plate. Spoon avocado into a bowl, mash with the lemon juice, and season with salt and pepper. Spread the mash on the patties. Boil 3 cups of water in a pan over high heat and reduce to simmer (don't boil). Crack an egg into a bowl and put it in the simmering water.

Poach for 2-3 minutes. Remove to a plate. Repeat with the remaining eggs. Top patties with eggs and sprinkle with chili flakes.

Per serving: Cal 378; Net Carbs 5g; Fat 23g; Protein 16g

Starter and Salad

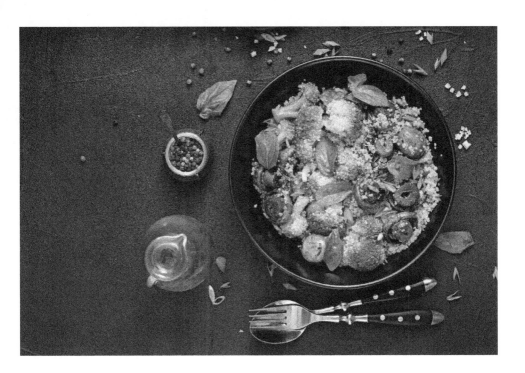

Saffron Cauli Rice with Fried Garlic

Ingredients for 4 servings

A pinch of saffron soaked in ¼-cup almond milk

2 tbsp olive oil

6 garlic cloves, sliced

1 tbsp butter

1 yellow onion, thinly sliced

2 cups cauli rice

¼ cup vegetable broth

Salt and black pepper to taste

2 tbsp chopped parsley

Directions and Total Time: approx. 35 minutes

Heat olive oil in a saucepan over medium heat and fry garlic until golden brown but not burned; set aside. Add butter to the saucepan and sauté onion for 3 minutes. Stir in cauli rice; remove the saffron from the milk and pour the milk and vegetable stock into the saucepan. Mix, cover, and cook for 5 minutes. Season with salt, black pepper, and parsley. Fluff the rice and dish into serving plates. Garnish with fried garlic and serve.

Per serving: Cal 91; Net Carbs 5.9g; Fat 6.6g; Protein 2g

Walnut Roasted Asparagus

Ingredients for 4 servings

2 tbsp olive oil

1 garlic clove, crushed

1 tbsp tamarind sauce

2 tbsp walnuts, chopped

1 ¼ lb asparagus, trimmed

3 tbsp tahini

2 tbsp balsamic vinegar

½ tbsp chili pepper, chopped

Directions and Total Time: approx. 20 minutes

Preheat oven to 350 F. In a bowl, mix olive oil, garlic, tamarind sauce, and walnuts. Lay asparagus on a baking tray and drizzle tamarind mixture all over.

Roast the veggies until tender and charred, 12 minutes. In a bowl, whisk tahini, balsamic vinegar, and chili pepper. Plate asparagus, drizzle with dressing, and serve.

Per serving: Cal 359; Net Carbs 8.4g; Fat 32g; Protein 9.6g

Crostini with Avocado

Ingredients for 4 servings

4 tbsp olive oil

2 avocados, chopped

¼ tsp garlic powder

¼ tsp onion powder

1 tbsp chopped parsley

1 lemon, zested and juiced

1 loaf zero carb bread, sliced

2 garlic cloves, halved

3 tbsp grated Parmesan

2 tbsp chopped toasted hazelnuts

Directions and Total Time: approx. 25 minutes

In a bowl, place 2 tbsp olive oil, avocado, garlic and onion powders, salt, pepper, parsley, zest, and juice and mix with a fork until smooth; set aside.

Heat a grill pan. Rub both sides of the bread slices with garlic and brush with remaining olive oil. Grill on both sides until crispy and golden. Spread the avocado mixture onto the crostini. Sprinkle with Parmesan cheese and hazelnuts. Drizzle with some more olive oil and serve.

Per serving: Cal 327; Net Carbs 3.9g; Fat 31g; Protein 3.6g

Speedy Slaw with Pecans

Ingredients for 4 servings

½ cup toasted pecans, chopped

2 cups broccoli slaw

1 red bell pepper, sliced

1 red onion, thinly sliced

2 tbsp chopped cilantro

2 tbsp flax seeds

1 tbsp red wine vinegar

2 tbsp olive oil

½ lemon, juiced

1 tsp Dijon mustard

2 tbsp mayonnaise

Salt and black pepper to taste

Directions and Total Time: approx. 20 minutes

In a bowl, combine broccoli slaw, bell pepper, red onion, cilantro, salt, and pepper. Mix in pecans and flax seeds. In a bowl, whisk vinegar, olive oil, lemon juice, mayonnaise, and mustard. Drizzle the dressing over the slaw and serve.

Per serving: Cal 310; Net Carbs 3.2g; Fat 31g; Protein 4.8g

Chili Broccoli Rabe with Sesame Seeds

Ingredients for 4 servings

3 cups broccoli rabe, chopped

1 tbsp melted butter

1 tbsp olive oil

1 garlic clove, minced

1 orange bell pepper, sliced

Salt and black pepper to taste

1 tbsp red chili flakes

Directions and Total Time: approx. 15 minutes

Cook broccoli in lightly salted water for 3 minutes or until softened; drain. Heat butter and olive oil in a skillet over medium heat and sauté garlic and bell pepper until softened, 5 minutes. Toss in broccoli. Sprinkle with flakes.

Per serving: Cal 68; Net Carbs 1.2g; Fat 6.4g; Protein 1.2g

Cheesy Zucchini Bake

Ingredients for 4 servings

3 large zucchinis, sliced

3 tbsp salted butter, melted

2 tbsp olive oil

1 garlic clove, minced

1 tsp dried thyme

¼ cup grated mozzarella

2/3 cup grated Parmesan

Directions and Total Time: approx. 25 minutes

Preheat oven to 350 F. Pour zucchini in a bowl; add in butter, olive oil, garlic, and thyme; toss to coat. Spread onto a baking dish and sprinkle with the mozzarella and Parmesan cheeses. Bake for 15 minutes. Serve warm.

Per serving: Cal 194; Net Carbs 3g; Fat 17.2g; Protein 7.4g

Soup and stews

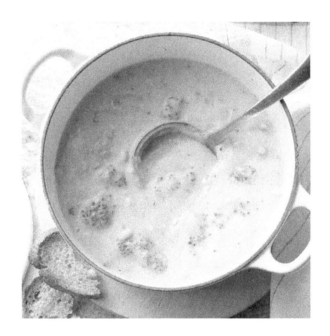

Creamy Chicken Soup

Ingredients for 4 servings

½ lb chicken breasts, chopped

3 tbsp butter, melted

4 cups chicken broth

4 tbsp chopped cilantro

⅓ cup buffalo sauce

4 oz cream cheese

Directions and Total Time: approx. 30 minutes

Blend butter, buffalo sauce, and cream cheese in a food processor until uniform and smooth. Transfer to a pot. Add the chicken to the pot, pour in the broth and cook for 20 minutes. Serve garnished with cilantro.

Per serving: Cal 406; Net Carbs 5g; Fat 29.5g, Protein 26g

Coconut Cream Pumpkin Soup

Ingredients for 4 servings

2 red onions, cut into wedges

2 garlic cloves

10 oz pumpkin, cubed

10 oz butternut squash, cubed

2 tbsp melted butter

8 oz butter

Salt and black pepper to taste

Juice of 1 lime

¾ cup mayonnaise

2 tbsp toasted pumpkin seeds

Directions and Total Time: approx. 55 minutes

Preheat oven to 400 F. Place onions, pumpkin, and butternut squash to a baking sheet and drizzle with melted butter. Season with salt and pepper. Roast for 30 minutes or until the veggies are golden brown and fragrant; transfer to a pot. Add in 2 cups water, bring to a boil, and cook for 15 minutes. Break the remaining butter in the pot and puree the vegetables until smooth. Stir in lime juice, and mayo. Serve garnished with toasted pumpkin seeds.

Per serving: Cal 643; Fat 57g; Net Carbs 9g; Protein 10g

Keto Reuben Soup

Ingredients for 6 servings

1 onion, diced

7 cups beef stock

1 tsp caraway seeds

2 celery stalks, diced

2 garlic cloves, minced

2 cups heavy cream

1 cup sauerkraut

1 lb corned beef, chopped

3 tbsp butter

1 ½ cups Swiss cheese, grated

Salt and black pepper to taste

Directions and Total Time: approx. 30 minutes

Melt butter in a large pot. Add in onion, garlic, and celery and fry for 3 minutes until tender. Pour the broth over and stir in sauerkraut, salt, caraway seeds, and pepper. Bring to a boil. Reduce the heat to low and add the corned beef. Cook for about 15 minutes. Stir in heavy cream and Swiss cheese and cook for 1 minute. Serve warm.

Per serving: Cal 450; Net Carbs 8g; Fat 37g, Protein 23g

Chorizo & Cauliflower Soup

Ingredients for 4 servings

1 cauliflower head, chopped

1 turnip, chopped

3 tbsp butter

1 chorizo sausage, sliced

2 cups chicken broth

1 small onion, chopped

2 cups water

Salt and black pepper to taste

Directions and Total Time: approx. 40 minutes

Melt 2 tbsp of butter in a pot. Stir in onion and sauté until soft and golden, 6 minutes. Add in cauliflower and turnip and cook for another 5 minutes. Pour in chicken broth. Bring to a boil and simmer for 20 minutes. Melt the remaining butter in a skillet. Add in chorizo and cook for 5 minutes. Blitz the soup with a hand blender until smooth. Adjust the seasonings. Serve topped with chorizo.

Per serving: Cal 251; Net Carbs 5.7g; Fat 19g, Protein 10g

Kale & Egg Soup

Ingredients for 4 servings

1 tbsp olive oil

2 tbsp butter

1 red onion, thinly sliced

1 carrot, chopped

3 garlic cloves, finely sliced

4 cups kale, chopped

1 lettuce head, chopped

4 cups vegetable stock

1 tbsp fresh dill

Salt and black pepper to taste

4 eggs

1 cup grated Parmesan cheese

Directions and Total Time: approx. 35 minutes

Warm oil and butter in a saucepan over medium heat and sauté onion, carrot, and garlic for 4 minutes. Stir in kale and lettuce and cook for 5 minutes. Pour in vegetable stock; bring to a boil. Reduce the heat and simmer for 10 minutes. With an immersion blender, puree the soup until smooth. Season with salt and pepper. Bring 1 cup of vinegared water to a boil in another saucepan. Create a whirlpool in the center using a wooden spoon. Allow water to almost settle back to normal and crack in an egg. Poach for 3 minutes, remove, and set aside in a plate. Repeat poaching the remaining eggs. Divide the soup into serving bowls. Top with poached eggs, sprinkle with dill and Parmesan cheese, and serve warm.

Lunch and dinner

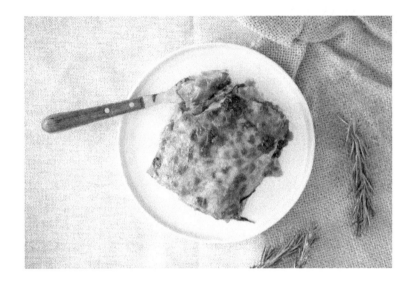

Seitan Kabobs with BBQ Sauce

Ingredients for 4 servings

10 oz seitan, cut into chunks

2 cups water

1 red onion, cut into chunks

1 red bell pepper, cut chunks

1 yellow bell pepper, chopped

2 tbsp olive oil

1 cup barbecue sauce

Salt and black pepper to taste

Directions and Total Time: approx. 30 min + marinating time : Bring water to a boil in a pot over medium heat, turn the heat off, and add seitan. Cover the pot and let the tempeh steam for 5 minutes; drain. Pour barbecue sauce in a bowl, add in the seitan, and toss to coat. Cover the bowl and marinate in the fridge for 2 hours.

Preheat grill to 350 F. Thread the seitan, yellow bell pepper, red bell pepper, and onion. Brush the grate of the grill with olive oil, place the skewers on it, and brush with barbecue sauce. Cook the kabobs for 3 minutes on each side while rotating and brushing with more barbecue sauce. Serve.

Per serving: Cal 228; Net Carbs 3.6g; Fat 15g; Protein 13g

Grilled Lamb Chops with Minty Sauce

Ingredients for 4 servings

8 lamb chops

2 tbsp favorite spice mix

¼ cup olive oil

1 tsp red pepper flakes

2 tbsp lemon juice

2 tbsp fresh mint

3 garlic cloves, pressed

2 tbsp lemon zest

¼ cup parsley

½ tsp smoked paprika

Directions and Total Time: approx. 25 minutes

Preheat grill to medium heat. Rub the lamb with oil and sprinkle with spices. Grill for 3 minutes per side. Whisk together the remaining oil, lemon juice and zest, mint, garlic, parsley, and paprika. Serve the chops with sauce.

Per serving: Cal 392; Net Carbs 0g; Fat 31g; Protein 29g

Grana Padano Roasted Cabbage

Ingredients for 4 servings

1 head green cabbage

4 tbsp melted butter

1 tsp garlic powder

Salt and black pepper to taste

1 cup grated Grana Padano

1 tbsp parsley, chopped

Directions and Total Time: approx. 30 minutes

Preheat oven to 400 F. Line a baking sheet with foil. Cut cabbage into wedges. Mix butter, garlic, salt, and pepper in a bowl. Brush the mixture on all sides of the wedges and sprinkle with some of Grana Padano cheese. Bake for 20 minutes. Sprinkle with remaining cheese and parsley.

Per serving: Cal 268; Net Carbs 4g; Fat 19g; Protein 17.5g

Pancetta Mashed Cauliflower

Ingredients for 4 servings

1 head cauliflower, leaves removed

6 slices pancetta

2 cups water

2 tbsp melted butter

½ cup buttermilk

¼ cup Colby cheese, grated

2 tbsp chopped chives

Directions and Total Time: approx. 40 minutes

Preheat oven to 350 F. Fry pancetta in a skillet over medium heat for 5 minutes. Let cool and crumble. Keep the pancetta fat. Boil cauli head in water in a pot for 7 minutes. Drain and put in a bowl. Add in butter and buttermilk and puree until smooth and creamy. Grease a casserole with the pancetta fat and spread the mash inside it. Sprinkle with colby cheese and place under the broiler for 4 minutes. Top with pancetta and chopped chives.

Per serving: Cal 312; Net Carbs 6g; Fat 25g; Protein 14g

Pancetta Wrapped Chicken Rolls

Ingredients for 4 servings

1 tbsp fresh chives, chopped

8 ounces blue cheese

1 lb chicken breasts, halved

12 pancetta slices

2 tomatoes, chopped

Salt and black pepper, to taste

Directions and Total Time: approx. 50 minutes

In a bowl, stir blue cheese, chives, tomatoes, pepper, and salt. Use a meat tenderizer to flatten the chicken breasts well, season with salt and pepper, and spread the cream cheese mixture on top. Roll them up and wrap in pancetta slices. Transfer to a greased baking dish and roast in the oven at 370 F for 30 minutes. Serve warm.

Per serving: Cal 623; Net Carbs 5g; Fat 48g; Protein 38g

Fish Taco Green Bowl with Red Cabbage

Ingredients for 4 servings

2 cups broccoli, riced

2 tsp ghee

4 tilapia fillets, cut into cubes

¼ tsp taco seasoning

Salt and chili pepper to taste

¼ head red cabbage, shredded

1 ripe avocado, chopped

1 tsp dill

Directions and Total Time: approx. 20 minutes

Sprinkle broccoli in a bowl with a little bit of water and microwave for 3 minutes. Fluff with a fork and set aside. Melt ghee in a skillet over medium heat, rub the tilapia with taco seasoning, salt, dill, and chili and fry until brown on all sides, 8 minutes in total; set aside. In 4 serving bowls, share the broccoli, cabbage, fish, and avocado. Serve.

Per serving: Cal 269; Net Carbs 4g; Fat 23g; Protein 16.5g

Herbed Veal Rack

Ingredients for 4 servings

12 ounces veal rack

2 fennel bulbs, sliced

Salt and black pepper to taste

3 tbsp olive oil

½ cup apple cider vinegar

1 tsp herbs de Provence

Directions and Total Time: approx. 50 minutes

Preheat oven to 400 F. In a bowl, mix fennel with 2 tbsp of oil and vinegar, toss to coat, and set to a baking dish. Season with herbs de Provence and bake for 15 minutes.

Sprinkle pepper and salt on the veal, place into an greased pan over medium-high heat, and cook for a couple of minutes. Place the veal in the baking dish with the fennel, and bake for 20 minutes. Serve.

Per serving: Cal 230; Net Carbs 5.2g; Fat 11g; Protein 19g

Cheese Scallops with Chorizo

Ingredients for 4 servings

2 tbsp ghee

16 fresh scallops

8 ounces chorizo, chopped

1 red bell pepper, sliced

1 cup red onions, chopped

1 cup Parmesan, grated

Directions and Total Time: approx. 15 minutes

Melt the ghee in a skillet and cook onion and bell pepper for 5 minutes. Add in chorizo and stir-fry for another 3 minutes; set aside. Season scallops with salt and pepper. Sear the scallops in the same skillet for 2 minutes on each side. Add the chorizo mixture back and warm through. Transfer to a serving platter and top with Parmesan cheese.

Per serving: Cal 491; Net Carbs 5g; Fat 32g; Protein 36g

Chicken Ham & Turnip Pasta

Ingredients for 4 servings

6 slices chicken ham, chopped

1 lb turnips, spiralized

1 tbsp smoked paprika

Salt and black pepper to taste

4 tbsp olive oil

Directions and Total Time: approx. 30 minutes

Preheat oven to 450 F. Pour turnips into a bowl and add in paprika, salt, and pepper; toss to coat. Spread the mixture on a greased baking sheet, scatter ham on top, and drizzle with olive oil. Bake for 10 minutes until golden brown.

Per serving: Cal 204; Net Carbs 1.6g; Fat 15g; Protein 10g

Kentucky Cauliflower with Mashed Parsnips

Ingredients for 6 servings

½ cup almond milk

¼ cup coconut flour

¼ tsp cayenne pepper

½ cup almond breadcrumbs

½ cup grated cheddar cheese

30 oz cauliflower florets

1 lb parsnips, quartered

3 tbsp melted butter

A pinch nutmeg

1 tsp cumin powder

1 cup coconut cream

2 tbsp sesame oil

Directions and Total Time: approx. 35 minutes Preheat oven to 425 F. Line a baking sheet with parchment paper. In a bowl, combine almond milk, coconut flour, and cayenne. In another bowl, mix breadcrumbs and cheddar cheese. Dip each cauliflower floret into the milk mixture, and then into the cheese mixture.

Place breaded cauliflower on the baking sheet and bake for 30 minutes, turning once. Pour 4 cups of slightly salted water in a pot and add in parsnips. Bring to boil and cook for 15 minutes. Drain and transfer to a bowl.

Add in melted butter, cumin, nutmeg, and coconut cream. Mash the ingredients using a potato mash. Spoon the mash into plates and drizzle with sesame oil. Serve with baked cauliflower.

__Poultry__

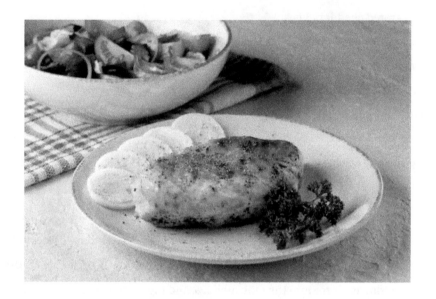

Hasselback Chicken

Ingredients for 6 servings

4 ounces cream cheese

3 oz mozzarella cheese slices

10 ounces spinach

⅓ cup shredded mozzarella

1 tbsp olive oil

⅔ cup tomato basil sauce

3 whole chicken breasts

Directions and Total Time: approx. 45 minutes

Preheat oven to 400 F. Mix cream cheese, shredded mozzarella cheese, and spinach and microwave the mixture until the cheese melts. Cut the chicken a couple of times horizontally. Stuff with the spinach mixture. Brush the top with olive oil. Place on a lined baking dish and bake in the oven for 25 minutes. Pour the tomato-basil sauce over and top with mozzarella slices. Return to the oven and bake for 5 more minutes. Serve warm.

Per serving: Cal 338; Net Carbs 2.5g; Fat 28g; Protein 37g

Spicy Chicken & Cheddar Pasta

Ingredients for 4 servings

2 (8 oz) packs shirataki fettuccine

4 chicken breasts

1 yellow onion, minced

3 garlic cloves, minced

1 tsp Italian seasoning

½ tsp garlic powder

¼ tsp red chili flakes

¼ tsp cayenne pepper

1 cup marinara sauce

1 cup grated mozzarella cheese

½ cup grated cheddar cheese

Salt and black pepper to taste

2 tbsp chopped parsley

Directions and Total Time: approx. 35 minutes: Boil 2 cups water in a pot over medium heat. Strain the shirataki pasta and rinse well under hot running water. Allow proper draining and pour the shirataki pasta into the boiling water. Cook for 3 minutes and strain again. Place a dry skillet and stir-fry the pasta until visibly dry, 1 to 2 minutes; set aside. Heat olive oil in a pot, season the chicken with salt and pepper, and cook for 10 minutes.

Cut into cubes and set aside. Add onion and garlic to the pan and cook for 3 minutes. Season with Italian seasoning, garlic powder, red chili flakes, and cayenne pepper. Stir in marinara sauce and simmer for 5 minutes. Return the chicken and shirataki fettuccine, mozzarella and cheddar cheeses. Stir until the cheeses melt. Garnish with parsley.

Chicken &Bacon Pie

Ingredients for 4 servings

¾ cup Greek yogurt

1 sweet onion, chopped

3 oz bacon, chopped

3 tbsp butter

1 carrot, chopped

3 garlic cloves, minced

Salt and black pepper, to taste

½ cup chicken stock

½ lb chicken breasts, cubed

¾ cup mozzarella, shredded

For the dough

¾ cup almond flour

2 tbsp cottage cheese

2 cups mozzarella, shredded

1 egg

1 tsp onion powder

1 tsp garlic powder

Directions and Total Time: approx. 55 minutes

Preheat oven to 370 F. Warm butter in a pan over medium heat and sauté onion, garlic, bacon, carrot, salt, and pepper for 5 minutes. Add in chicken and cook for

3 minutes. Stir in yogurt and stock and cook for 7 minutes. Stir in ¾ cup mozzarella cheese; set aside. Microwave mozzarella and cottage cheeses from the dough ingredients for 1 minute. Stir in garlic powder, almond flour, onion powder, and egg. Knead the dough well, split into 4 pieces, and flatten each into a circle. Set the chicken mixture into 4 ramekins, top each with a dough circle, and bake for 25 minutes.

Per serving: Cal 503; Net Carbs 5.6g; Fat 31g; Protein 41g

Kale & Tomato Chicken with Linguine

Ingredients for 4 servings

1 cup grated Parmigiano-Reggiano cheese for serving

4 chicken thighs, cut into 1-inch pieces

1 cup cherry tomatoes, halved

1 cup shredded mozzarella

1 egg yolk

3 tbsp olive oil

Salt and black pepper to taste

1 yellow onion, chopped

4 garlic cloves, minced

½ cup chicken broth

2 cups baby kale, chopped

2 tbsp pine nuts for topping

Directions and Total Time: approx. 45 min + chilling time

Microwave mozzarella cheese for 2 minutes. Take out the bowl and allow cooling for 1 minute. Mix in egg yolk until well-combined. Lay a parchment paper on a flat surface, pour the cheese mixture on top and cover with another parchment paper. Flatten the dough into 1/8-inch thickness. Take off the parchment paper and cut the dough into linguine strands. Place in a bowl and refrigerate overnight. Bring 2 cups water to a boil and add in keto linguine. Cook for 1 minute and drain; set aside.

Heat olive oil in a pot, season the chicken with salt and pepper, and sear it for 6-8 minutes; set aside. Add onion and garlic to the pot and cook for 3 minutes. Mix in tomatoes and broth and return the chicken; cook until the liquid reduces by half, about 10 minutes. Stir in kale for 5 minutes. Divide linguine between serving plates, pour in the chicken/kale mixture and sprinkle with Parmigianino-Reggiano cheese. Garnish with pine nuts.

Per serving: Cal 740; Net Carbs 6g; Fats 52g; Protein 51g

One-Pot Mustard Chicken with Pancetta

Ingredients for 4 servings

3 oz smoked pancetta, chopped

5 tbsp Dijon mustard

1 fennel bulb, sliced

1 onion, chopped

2 tbsp olive oil

1 cup chicken stock

1 pound chicken breasts

¼ tsp sweet paprika

Directions and Total Time: approx. 40 minutes

Put mustard in a bowl and add in paprika, salt, and pepper; stir to combine. Massage the mixture onto all sides of the chicken. Warm 1 tbsp olive oil in a pot over medium heat and cook the chicken for 3 minutes per side or until golden; set aside. To the same pot, add the remaining olive oil and cook pancetta, onion, and fennel for 5 minutes. Return chicken, pour in stock, and simmer for 20 minutes.

Per serving: Cal 368; Net Carbs 2.5g; Fat 24g; Protein 28g

Creamy Greens & Chicken in a Skillet

Ingredients for 4 servings

1 pound chicken thighs

2 tbsp coconut oil

2 tbsp coconut flour

2 carp dark leafy greens

1 tsp oregano

1 cup heavy cream

1 cup chicken broth

2 tbsp butter, melted

Directions and Total Time: approx. 35 minutes

Melt coconut oil in a skillet over medium heat and brown the chicken on all sides for 7-9 minutes; set aside. Melt butter in the same skillet and whisk in the coconut flour. Whisk in the chicken broth and bring to a boil. Stir in oregano, leafy greens, and heavy cream for 1 minute. Add in the thighs back and cook for an additional 10 minutes.

Per serving: Cal 446; Net Carbs 2.6g; Fat 38g; Protein 18g

Crispy Lemon & Thyme Chicken

Ingredients for 4 servings

8 chicken thighs

1 tsp salt

2 tbsp lemon juice

1 tsp lemon zest

2 tbsp olive oil

1 tbsp chopped thyme

¼ tsp black pepper

1 garlic cloves, minced

Directions and Total Time: approx. 20 min + chilling time

Combine all ingredients in a bowl. Cover and place to marinate in the fridge for 1 hour. Heat a skillet over medium heat. Add the marinated chicken and their juices and cook until crispy, 7 minutes per side. Serve warm.

Per serving: Cal 477; Net Carbs 1.2g; Fat 32g; Protein 31g

Roasted Chicken with Brussel Sprouts

Ingredients for 6 servings

5-pound whole chicken

1 bunch oregano

1 bunch thyme

1 tbsp parsley

1 tbsp olive oil

2 pounds Brussels sprouts

1 lemon

4 tbsp butter

Directions and Total Time: approx. 65 minutes

Preheat oven to 450 F. Stuff the chicken with oregano, thyme, and lemon. Make sure the wings are tucked over and behind. Roast in the oven for 15 minutes. Reduce the heat to 325 F and cook for 20 minutes. Spread the butter over the chicken and sprinkle with parsley. Add the Brussels sprouts. Return to oven and bake for 25 more minutes. Let sit for 10 minutes before carving. Serve.

Per serving: Cal 430; Net Carbs 5.1g; Fat 32g; Protein 30g

Braised Chicken with Tomatoes & Eggplants

Ingredients for 4 servings

2 cups canned tomatoes

2 green onions, chopped

2 cloves garlic, minced

2 tbsp butter

1 lb chicken thighs

Salt and black pepper to taste

1 cup eggplants, cubed

2 tbsp fresh basil, chopped

Directions and Total Time: approx. 45 minutes

Season chicken with salt and pepper. Melt butter in a saucepan and fry chicken, skin side down for 4 minutes. Flip and cook for another 2 minutes; remove to a plate. In the same saucepan, sauté garlic and green onions for 3 minutes. Add in eggplants and cook for 5 minutes. Stir in tomatoes and cook for 10 minutes. Season the sauce with salt and pepper, stir, and add back the chicken. Simmer for 15 minutes. Garnish with fresh basil and serve.

Per serving: Cal 366; Net Carbs 6.9g; Fat 25g; Protein 21g

Beef

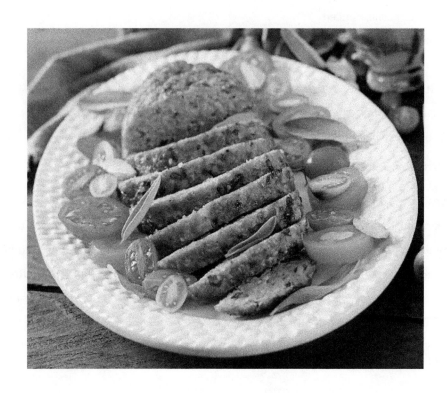

Spicy Enchilada Beef Stuffed Peppers

Ingredients for 6 servings

6 bell peppers, deseeded

1 ½ tbsp olive oil

3 tbsp butter, softened

½ white onion, chopped

3 cloves garlic, minced

2 ½ lb ground beef

3 tsp enchilada seasoning

1 cup cauliflower rice

¼ cup grated cheddar cheese

Sour cream for serving

Directions and Total Time: approx. 70 minutes

Preheat oven to 400 F. Melt butter in a skillet over medium heat and sauté onion and garlic for 3 minutes. Stir in beef, enchilada seasoning, salt, and pepper. Cook for 10 minutes. Mix in the cauli rice until well incorporated.

Spoon the mixture into the peppers, top with the cheddar cheese, and put the stuffed peppers in a greased baking dish. Bake for 40 minutes. Drop generous dollops of sour cream on the peppers and serve.

Per serving: Cal 409; Net Carbs 4g; Fat 21g; Protein 45g

Spicy Beef Lettuce Wraps

Ingredients for 4 servings

1 lb chuck steak, sliced thinly against the grain

3 tbsp ghee, divided

1 large white onion, chopped

2 garlic cloves, minced

1 jalapeño pepper, chopped

2 tsp red curry powder

1 cup cauliflower rice

8 small lettuce leaves

¼ cup sour cream for topping

Directions and Total Time: approx. 20 minutes

Melt 2 tbsp of ghee in a large deep skillet; season the beef and cook until brown and cooked within, 10 minutes; set aside. Sauté the onion for 3 minutes. Pour in garlic, salt, pepper, and jalapeño and cook for 1 minute.

Add the remaining ghee, curry powder, and beef. Cook for 5 minutes and stir in the cauliflower rice. Sauté until adequately mixed and the cauliflower is slightly softened, 2 to 3 minutes. Adjust the taste with salt and black pepper.

Lay out the lettuce leaves on a lean flat surface and spoon the beef mixture onto the middle part of them, 3 tbsp per leaf. Top with sour cream, wrap the leaves, and serve.

Per serving: Cal 298; Net Carbs 3.3g; Fat 18g; Protein 27g

Sunday Beef Sausage Pizza

Ingredients for 4 servings

2 tbsp cream cheese, softened

6 oz shredded cheese

¾ cup almond flour

1 egg

1 tsp plain vinegar

2 tbsp butter

8 oz ground beef sausage

¼ cup tomato sauce

½ tsp dried basil

4 ½ oz shredded mozzarella

Directions and Total Time: approx. 45 minutes

Preheat oven to 400 F. Line a pizza pan with parchment paper. Melt cream and mozzarella cheeses in a skillet while stirring until evenly combined. Turn the heat off and mix in almond flour, egg, and vinegar. Let cool slightly.

Flatten the mixture onto the pizza pan. Cover with another parchment paper and using a rolling pin, smoothen the dough into a circle. Take off the parchment paper on top, prick the dough all over with a fork and bake for 10 to 15 minutes until golden brown.

While the crust bakes, melt butter in a skillet over and fry sausage until brown, 8 minutes. Turn the heat off. Spread the tomato sauce on the crust, top with basil, meat, and mozzarella cheese, and return to the oven. Bake for 12 minutes. Remove the pizza, slice, and serve warm.

Per serving: Cal 361; Net Carbs 0.8g; Fat 21g; Protein 37g

Peanut Zucchini & Beef Pad Thai

Ingredients for 4 servings

2 ½ lb chuck steak, sliced thinly against the grain

1 tsp crushed red pepper flakes

1 tsp freshly pureed garlic

¼ tsp freshly ground ginger

Salt and black pepper to taste

2 tbsp peanut oil

3 large eggs, lightly beaten

1/3 cup beef broth

3 ¼ tbsp peanut butter

2 tbsp tamari sauce

1 tbsp white vinegar

½ cup chopped green onions

2 garlic cloves, minced

4 zucchinis, spiralized

½ cup bean sprouts

½ cup crushed peanuts

Directions and Total Time: approx. 35 minutes

In a bowl, combine garlic puree, ginger, salt, and pepper. Add in beef and toss to coat. Heat peanut oil in a deep skillet and cook the beef for 12 minutes; transfer to a plate. Pour the eggs to the skillet and scramble for 1 minute; set aside. Reduce the heat and combine broth, peanut butter, tamari sauce, vinegar, green onions, minced garlic, and red pepper flakes. Mix until adequately combined and simmer for 3 minutes. Stir in beef, zucchini, bean sprouts, and eggs. Cook for 1 minute. Garnish with peanuts.

Per serving: Cal 425; Net Carbs 3.3g; Fat 40g; Protein 70g

Lemon & Spinach Cheeseburgers

Ingredients for 4 servings

1 large tomato, sliced into 4 pieces and deseeded

1 lb ground beef

½ cup chopped cilantro

1 lemon, zested and juiced

Salt and black pepper to taste

1 tsp garlic powder

2 tbsp hot chili puree

16 large spinach leaves

4 tbsp mayonnaise

1 medium red onion, sliced

¼ cup grated Parmesan

1 avocado, halved, sliced

Directions and Total Time: approx. 15 minutes

Preheat the grill on high heat. In a bowl, add beef, cilantro, lemon zest, juice, salt, pepper, garlic powder, and chili puree. Mix the ingredients until evenly combined. Make 4 patties from the mixture. Grill for 3 minutes on each side. Transfer to a serving plate. Lay 2 spinach leaves side to side in 4 portions on a clean flat surface. Place a beef patty on each and spread 1 tbsp of mayo on top. Add a slice of tomato and onion, sprinkle with some Parmesan cheese, and place avocado on top. Cover with 2 pieces of spinach leaves each. Serve the burgers with cream cheese sauce.

Per serving: Cal 310; Net Carbs 6.5g; Fat 16g; Protein 29g

Herby Beef Meatballs

Ingredients for 4 servings

1 lb ground beef

1 red onion, finely chopped

2 red bell peppers, chopped

2 garlic cloves, minced

2 tbsp melted butter

1 tsp dried basil

2 tbsp tamari sauce

Salt and black pepper to taste

1 tbsp dried rosemary

1 tbsp olive oil

Directions and Total Time: approx. 30 minutes

Preheat the oven to 400 F. In a bowl, mix beef, onion, bell peppers, garlic, butter, basil, tamari sauce, salt, pepper, and rosemary. Form 1-inch meatballs from the mixture and place on a greased baking sheet. Drizzle olive oil over the beef and bake in the oven for 20 minutes or until the meatballs brown on the outside. Serve garnished with scallions and topped with ranch dressing.

Per serving: Cal 618; Net Carbs 2.5g; Fat 33g; Protein 74g

Keto Burgers

Ingredients for 4 servings

1 pound ground beef

½ tsp onion powder

½ tsp garlic powder

2 tbsp ghee

1 tsp Dijon mustard

4 zero carb burger buns

¼ cup mayonnaise

1 tsp Sriracha sauce

4 tbsp coleslaw

Salt and black pepper to taste

Directions and Total Time: approx. 15 minutes

Mix together beef, onion powder, garlic powder, and mustard in a bowl. Create 4 burgers. Melt ghee in a skillet and cook the burgers for 3 minutes per side. Serve on buns topped with mayonnaise, sriracha sauce, and coleslaw.

Per serving: Cal 664; Net Carbs 7.9g; Fat 55g; Protein 39g

Polish Beef Tripe

Ingredients for 6 servings

1 ½ lb beef tripe

4 cups buttermilk

Salt and black pepper to taste

1 parsnip, chopped

2 tsp marjoram

3 tbsp butter

2 large onions, sliced

3 tomatoes, diced

Directions and Total Time: approx. 30 min + cooling time

Put tripe in a bowl and cover with buttermilk. Refrigerate for 3 hours. Remove from buttermilk and season with salt and pepper. Heat 2 tablespoons butter in a skillet and brown the tripe for 6 minutes in total; set aside. Add the remaining butter and sauté onions for 3 minutes. Include tomatoes and parsnip and cook for 10-15 minutes. Put the tripe in the sauce and cook for 3 minutes. Serve warm.

Per serving: Cal 342, Net Carbs 1g, Fat 27g, Protein 22g

Pork

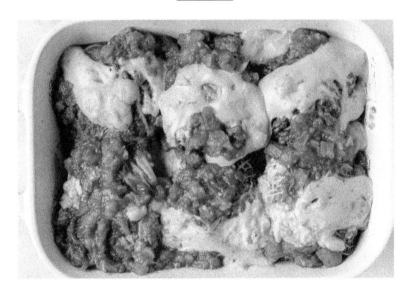

Yummy Spareribs in Béarnaise Sauce

Ingredients for 4 servings

3 tbsp butter, melted

4 egg yolks, beaten

2 tbsp chopped tarragon

2 tsp white wine vinegar

½ tsp onion powder

Salt and black pepper to taste

4 tbsp olive oil

2 lb spareribs, divided into 16

Directions and Total Time: approx. 30 minutes

In a bowl, whisk butter gradually into the egg yolks until evenly mixed. In another bowl, combine tarragon, white wine vinegar, and onion powder. Mix into the egg mixture and season with salt and black pepper; reserve the sauce.

Warm the olive oil in a skillet over medium heat. Season the spareribs on both sides with salt and pepper. Cook in the oil on both sides until brown, 12 minutes. Divide the spareribs between plates and serve with béarnaise sauce to the side along with some braised asparagus.

Per serving: Cal 878; Net Carbs 1g; Fat 78g; Protein 41g

Italian Pork with Capers

Ingredients for 4 servings

1 ½ lb thin cut pork chops, boneless

½ lemon, juiced + 1 lemon, sliced

Salt and black pepper to taste

1 tbsp avocado oil

3 tbsp butter

2 tbsp capers

1 cup beef broth

2 tbsp chopped parsley

Directions and Total Time: approx. 30 minutes

Heat avocado oil in a skillet and cook pork chops on both sides until brown, 14 minutes. Transfer to a plate and cover to keep warm. Melt butter in the skillet and cook capers until sizzling; keep stirring to avoid burning, 3 minutes. Pour in broth and lemon juice, use a spatula to scrape any bits stuck at the bottom, and boil until the sauce reduces by half. Add back the pork, arrange lemon slices on top, and sprinkle with 1 tbsp parsley. Simmer for 3 minutes. Serve the chops garnished with the remaining parsley.

Per serving: Cal 341; Net Carbs 0.8g; Fat 18g; Protein 40g

Pork Bake with Cottage Cheese & Olives

Ingredients for 4 servings

½ cup cottage cheese, crumbled

2 tbsp avocado oil

1 ½ lb ground pork

¼ cup sliced Kalamata olives

2 garlic cloves, minced

½ cup marinara sauce

1 ¼ cups heavy cream

Directions and Total Time: approx. 40 minutes

Preheat oven to 400 F. Grease a casserole dish with cooking spray. Heat avocado oil in a deep skillet, add the ground pork, and cook until brown, 10 minutes. Stir frequently and break any lumps that form. Spread the pork on the bottom of the casserole. Scatter olives, cottage cheese, and garlic on top. In a bowl, mix marinara sauce and heavy cream and pour all over the meat. Bake until the top is bubbly and lightly brown, 20-25 minutes. Serve.

Per serving: Cal 451; Net Carbs 1.5g; Fat 30g; Protein 40g

Parmesan & Pimiento Pork Meatballs

Ingredients for 4 servings

¼ cup chopped pimientos

1/3 cup mayonnaise

3 tbsp softened cream cheese

1 tsp paprika powder

1 pinch cayenne pepper

1 tbsp Dijon mustard

4 oz grated Parmesan cheese

1 ½ lb ground pork

1 large egg

2 tbsp olive oil, for frying

Directions and Total Time: approx. 30 minutes

In a bowl, mix pimientos, mayonnaise, cream cheese, paprika, cayenne pepper, mustard, Parmesan cheese, ground pork, and egg. Mix and form large meatballs. Heat olive oil in a non-stick skillet and fry the meatballs in batches on both sides until brown, 10 minutes in total. Transfer to a plate and serve on a bed of leafy green salad.

Per serving: Cal 485; Net Carbs 6.8g; Fat 30g; Protein 47g

Pork & Pecan in Camembert Bake

Ingredients for 4 servings

9 oz whole Camembert cheese

½ lb boneless pork chops, cut into small cubes

3 tbsp olive oil

2 oz pecans

1 garlic clove, minced

1 tbsp chopped parsley

Directions and Total Time: approx. 30 minutes

Preheat oven to 400 F. While the cheese is in its box, using a knife, score around the top and side of about a ¼-inch and take off the top layer of the skin. Place the cheese on a baking tray and melt in the oven for 10 minutes.

Meanwhile, heat olive oil in a skillet and fry the pork until brown on all sides, 12 minutes. Transfer to a bowl and add pecans, garlic, and parsley. Spoon the pork mixture onto the melted cheese and bake in the oven for 10 minutes until the cheese softens and nuts toast.

Per serving: Cal 452; Net Carbs 0.2g; Fat 38g; Protein 27g

Zucchini & Tomato Pork Omelet

Ingredients for 4 servings

3 zucchinis, halved lengthwise

4 tbsp olive oil

1 garlic clove, crushed

1 small plum tomato, diced

2 tbsp chopped scallions

1 tsp dried basil

1 tsp cumin powder

1 tsp smoked paprika

1 lb ground pork

3 large eggs, beaten

3 tsp crushed pork rinds

1/3 cup chopped cilantro

Directions and Total Time: approx. 50 minutes

Preheat a grill to medium. Drizzle the zucchinis with some olive oil and place them on the grill; broil until brown, 5 minutes. Heat remaining olive oil in a skillet and sauté garlic, tomato, and scallions for 8 minutes. Mix in basil, cumin, and paprika. Add and brown the ground pork for 10 minutes; reserve. Spread the pork mixture onto the grilled zucchini slices; flatten the mixture. Transfer to a greased baking dish. Divide the eggs between the zucchinis and place in preheated to 380 F oven. Cook until set, 8 minutes. Sprinkle pork rinds and cilantro on top and serve.

Per serving: Cal 332; Net Carbs 1.1g; Fat 22g; Protein 30g

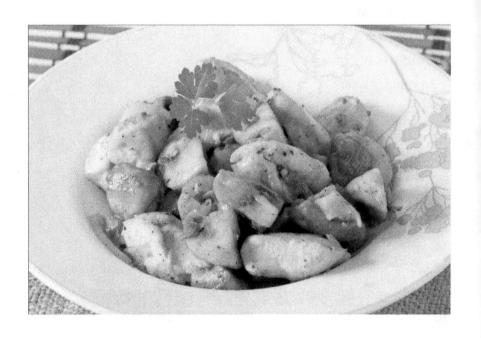

Buttered Pork Chops with Lemon Asparagus

Ingredients for 4 servings

7 tbsp butter

4 pork chops

Salt and black pepper to taste

4 tbsp butter, softened

2 garlic cloves, minced

1 lb asparagus, trimmed

1 tbsp dried cilantro

1 small lemon, juice

Directions and Total Time: approx. 30 minutes

Melt 3 tbsp of butter in a skillet over medium heat. Season pork chops with salt and pepper and fry on both sides until brown, 10 minutes in total; set aside. Melt the remaining butter in the skillet and sauté garlic until fragrant, 1 minute. Add in asparagus and cook until slightly softened with some crunch, 4 minutes. Add cilantro and lemon juice and toss to coat well. Serve the asparagus with the pork chops.

Per serving: Cal 538; Net Carbs 1.2g; Fat 38g; Protein 42g

Avocado & Green Bean Pork Sauté

Ingredients for 4 servings

4 tbsp avocado oil

4 pork shoulder chops

2 tbsp avocado oil

1 ½ cups green beans

2 large avocados, chopped

Salt and black pepper to taste

6 green onions, chopped

1 tbsp chopped parsley

Directions and Total Time: approx. 30 minutes

Heat avocado oil in a skillet, season pork with salt and pepper, and fry until brown, 12 minutes; set aside. To the same skillet, sauté green beans until sweating and slightly softened, 10 minutes. Mix in avocados and half of green onions for 2 minutes. Dish into plates, garnish with the remaining onions and parsley, and serve with pork chops.

Per serving: Cal 557; Net Carbs 1.9g; Fat 36g; Protein 43g

Seafood

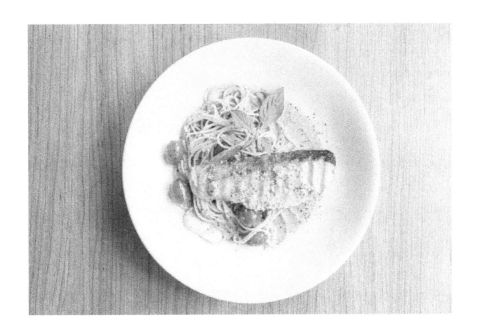

Teriyaki Salmon with Steamed Broccoli

Ingredients for 4 servings

¼ cup grated Pecorino Romano cheese + some more

4 salmon fillets

½ cup teriyaki sauce

1 bunch of broccoli rabe

Salt and black pepper to taste

Directions and Total Time: approx. 30 min + chilling time

Cover the salmon with the teriyaki sauce and refrigerate for 30 minutes. Steam the broccoli rabe for 4-5 minutes until tender. Season with salt and pepper and set aside.Preheat oven to 400 F. Remove the salmon from the fridge and place in a greased baking dish. Bake in the oven for 14-16 minutes. Serve with steamed broccoli rabe.

Per serving: Cal 354; Net Carbs 4g; Fat 17g; Protein 28g

Baked Salmon with Pistachio Crust

Ingredients for 4 servings

4 salmon fillets

¼ cup mayonnaise

½ cup ground pistachios

1 chopped shallot

2 tsp lemon zest

1 tbsp olive oil

A pinch of pepper

1 cup heavy cream

Directions and Total Time: approx. 35 minutes

Preheat oven to 375 F. Spread mayonnaise on the fillets. Coat with ground pistachios. Place in a lined baking dish and bake for 15 minutes. Heat the olive oil in a saucepan and sauté shallot for 3 minutes. Stir in heavy cream and lemon zest. Bring to a boil and cook until thickened. Pour the sauce over the salmon and serve.

Per serving: Cal 563; Net Carbs 6g; Fat 47g; Protein 34g

Party Smoked Salmon Balls

Ingredients for 6 servings

12 oz sliced smoked salmon, finely chopped

1 parsnip, cooked and mashed

Salt and chili pepper to taste

4 tbsp olive oil

2 eggs, beaten

2 tbsp pesto sauce

1 tbsp pork rinds, crushed

Directions and Total Time: approx. 30 minutes

In a bowl, add the salmon, eggs, pesto sauce, pork rinds, salt, and chili pepper. Mix well and make 6 compact balls. Heat olive oil in a skillet over medium heat and fry the balls for 3 minutes on each side until golden brown. Remove to a wire rack to cool. Serve warm.

Per serving: Cal 254; Net Carbs 4.3g; Fat 18g; Protein 17g

Salmon Caesar Salad with Poached Eggs

Ingredients for 4 servings

½ cup chopped smoked salmon

2 tbsp heinz low carb caesar dressing

3 cups water

8 eggs

2 cups torn romaine lettuce

4 pancetta slices

Directions and Total Time: approx. 15 minutes

Boil water in a pot over medium heat. Crack each egg into a small bowl and gently slide into the water. Poach for 2-3 minutes, remove, and transfer to a plate. Poach the remaining eggs. Put the pancetta in a skillet and fry for 6 minutes, turning once. Allow cooling and chop into small pieces. Toss the lettuce, smoked salmon, pancetta, and caesar dressing in a salad bowl. Top with the eggs.

Per serving: Cal 260; Net Carbs 5g; Fat 21g; Protein 8g

Vegan and vegetarian

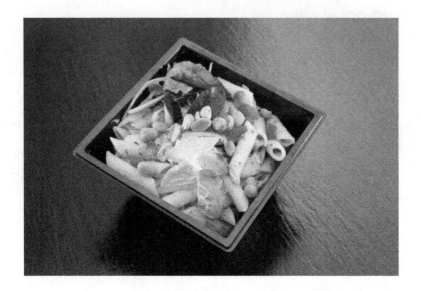

Olive & Avocado Zoodles

Ingredients for 4 servings

¼ cup chopped sun-dried tomatoes

4 zucchini, spiralized

½ cup pesto

2 avocados, sliced

1 cup kalamata olives, chopped

¼ cup chopped basil

2 tbsp olive oil

Directions and Total Time: approx. 15 minutes

Heat 1 tbsp olive oil in a pan over medium heat. Add zoodles and cook for 4 minutes. Transfer to a plate. Stir in 1 tbsp olive oil, pesto, basil, tomatoes, and olives. Top with avocado slices. Serve.

Per serving: Cal 449; Net Carbs 8.4g; Fat 42g; Protein 6g

Chia Seed Ice Cream

Ingredients for 4 servings

2 tbsp chia seeds

Juice and zest of 3 limes

1/3 cup erythritol

1¾ cups coconut cream

¼ tsp vanilla extract

Directions and Total Time: approx. 10 minutes

In a bowl, combine avocado pulp chia seeds, lime juice and zest, erythritol, coconut cream, and vanilla extract and mix well. Pour the mixture into an ice cream maker and freeze. When ready, remove and scoop the ice cream into dessert cups. Serve immediately.

Per serving: Cal 260; Net Carbs 4g; Fat 25g; Protein 4g

White Egg Tex Mex Pizza

Ingredients for 2 servings

4 eggs

2 tbsp water

1 Jalapeno pepper, diced

2 oz Monterey Jack, shredded

2 tbsp chopped green onions

¼ cup Alfredo sauce

¼ tsp cumin

2 tbsp olive oil

Directions and Total Time: approx. 17 minutes

Preheat the oven to 350 F. Heat olive oil in a skillet. Whisk the eggs along with water and cumin; pour into the skillet and cook until set. Top with alfredo sauce and jalapeno pepper. Sprinkle green onions and cheese over. Place in the oven and bake for 5 minutes. Serve warm.

Per serving: Cal 591; Net Carbs 2g; Fat 55g; Protein 22g

Quick Grilled Cheddar Cheese

Ingredients for 2 servings

4 eggs

1 tsp baking powder

3 tbsp butter

3 tbsp almond flour

2 tbsp psyllium husk powder

4 oz cheddar cheese

Directions and Total Time: approx. 15 minutes

Whisk together all ingredients, except for 1 tbsp butter and cheddar cheese. Microwave for 90 seconds. Flip the "bun" over and cut in half. Place the cheddar on one half of the bun and top with the other. Melt the remaining butter in a skillet. Add the sandwich and grill until the cheese is melted and the bun is crispy. Serve.

Per serving: Cal 623; Net Carbs 6.1g; Fat 51g; Protein 25g

Enchilada Vegetarian Pasta

Ingredients for 4 servings

1 cup shredded mozzarella

1 cup chopped bell peppers

1 egg yolk

1 tsp olive oil

2 garlic cloves, minced

2 cups enchilada sauce

1 tsp cumin powder

½ tsp smoked paprika

1 tsp chili powder

Salt and black pepper to taste

¾ cup chopped green onions

1 avocado, pitted, sliced

Directions and Total Time: approx. 20 min + chilling time: Microwave mozzarella cheese for 2 minutes. Take out the bowl and allow cooling for 1 minute. Mix in egg yolk until well-combined. Lay a parchment paper on a flat surface, pour the cheese mixture on top and cover with another parchment paper. Flatten the dough into 1/8-inch thickness. Take off the parchment paper and cut the dough into penne-size pieces. Place in a bowl and refrigerate overnight. Bring 2 cups water to a boil in medium saucepan and add the keto penne. Cook for 1 minute and drain; set aside. Heat olive oil in a skillet and sauté garlic for 30 seconds. Mix in enchilada sauce, cumin, paprika, chili powder, bell peppers, salt, and pepper. Cook for 5 minutes. Mix in pasta. Top with green onions and avocado.

Per serving: Cal 151; Net Carbs 3.3g; Fats 8g; Prote

Pepper & Broccoli with Zucchini Spaghetti

Ingredients for 4 servings

1 head broccoli, cut into florets

1 cup sliced mixed bell peppers

2 tbsp olive oil

4 zucchinis, spiralized

4 shallots, finely chopped

Salt and black pepper to taste

2 garlic cloves, minced

¼ tsp red pepper flakes

1 cup chopped kale

2 tbsp balsamic vinegar

½ lemon, juiced

1 cup grated Parmesan cheese

Directions and Total Time: approx. 20 minutes

Heat oil in a skillet and sauté broccoli, bell peppers, and shallots until softened, 7 minutes. Mix in garlic, and red pepper flakes and cook until fragrant, 30 seconds. Stir in kale and zucchini spaghetti; cook until tender, 3 minutes. Mix in vinegar and lemon juice and adjust the taste with salt and pepper. Garnish with Parmesan cheese and serve.

Per serving: Cal 199; Net Carbs 5.9g; Fats 13g; Protein 9g

Herby Mushroom Pizza

Ingredients for 4 servings

2 medium cremini mushrooms, sliced

2 ½ cups grated mozzarella

½ cup grated Parmesan cheese

2 tbsp cream cheese, softened

½ cup almond flour

1 egg, beaten

1 tsp olive oil

1 garlic clove, minced

½ cup tomato sauce

1 tsp erythritol

1 tsp dried oregano

1 tsp dried basil

½ tsp paprika

Salt and black pepper to taste

6 black olives, sliced

Directions and Total Time: approx. 45 minutes

Preheat oven to 390 F. Line a pizza pan with parchment paper. Microwave 2 cups mozzarella cheese and 2 tbsp cream cheese for 1 minute. Mix in almond meal and egg. Spread the mixture on the pizza pan and bake for 5 minutes; set aside. Heat olive oil in a skillet and sauté mushrooms and garlic until softened, 5 minutes. Mix in tomato sauce, erythritol, oregano, basil, paprika, salt, and pepper. Cook for

2 minutes. Spread the sauce on the crust, top with the remaining mozzarella and Parmesan cheeses and olives. Bake for 15 minutes. Slice and serve.

Per serving: Cal 203; Net Carbs 2.6g; Fats 8g; Protein 23g

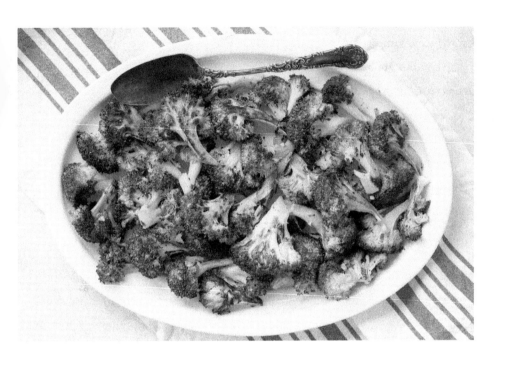

Snacks and side dish

Cheddar Bacon & Celeriac Bake

Ingredients for 4 servings

6 bacon slices, chopped

3 tbsp butter

3 garlic cloves, minced

3 tbsp almond flour

2 cups coconut cream

1 cup chicken broth

Salt and black pepper to taste

1 lb celeriac, peeled and sliced

2 cups shredded cheddar

¼ cup chopped scallions

Directions and Total Time: approx. 50 minutes

Preheat oven to 400 F. Add bacon to a skillet and fry over medium heat until brown and crispy. Spoon onto a plate. Melt butter in the same skillet and sauté garlic for 1 minute. Mix in almond flour and cook for another minute. Whisk in coconut cream, chicken broth, salt, and pepper. Simmer for 5 minutes. Spread a layer of the sauce in a greased casserole dish and arrange a layer celeriac on top. Cover with more sauce, top with some bacon and cheddar cheese, and scatter scallions on top. Repeat the layering process until the ingredients are exhausted. Bake for 35 minutes. Let rest for a few minutes and serve.

Per serving: Cal 981; Net Carbs 20g; Fat 86g; Protein 28g

Chicken Ham with Mini Bell Peppers

Ingredients for 4 servings

12 mini green bell peppers, halved and deseeded

4 slices chicken ham, chopped

1 tbsp chopped parsley

8 oz cream cheese

½ tbsp hot sauce

2 tbsp melted butter

1 cup shredded Gruyere

Directions and Total Time: approx. 30 minutes

Preheat oven to 400 F. Place peppers in a greased baking dish and set aside. In a bowl, combine chicken ham, parsley, cream cheese, hot sauce, and butter. Spoon the mixture into the peppers and sprinkle Gruyere cheese on top. Bake until the cheese melts, about 20 minutes. Serve.

Per serving: Cal 408; Net Carbs 4g; Fat 32g; Protein 19g

Crispy Baked Cheese Asparagus

Ingredients for 4 servings

1 cup grated Pecorino Romano cheese

4 slices Serrano ham, chopped

2 lb asparagus, stalks trimmed

¾ cup coconut cream

3 garlic cloves, minced

1 cup crushed pork rinds

1 cup grated mozzarella

½ tsp sweet paprika

Directions and Total Time: approx. 40 minutes

Preheat oven to 400 F. Arrange asparagus on a greased baking dish and pour coconut cream on top. Scatter the garlic, serrano ham, and pork rinds on top and sprinkle with Pecorino cheese, mozzarella cheese, and paprika. Bake until the cheese melts and is golden and asparagus tender, 30 minutes. Serve warm.

Per serving: Cal 361; Net Carbs 15g; Fat 21g; Protein 32g

Easy Bacon & Cheese Balls

Ingredients for 4 servings

7 bacon slices

6 oz cream cheese

6 oz shredded Gruyere cheese

2 tbsp butter, softened

½ tsp red chili flakes

Directions and Total Time: approx. 30 minutes

Put bacon in a skillet and fry over medium heat until crispy, 5 minutes. Transfer to a plate to cool and cruble it. Pour the bacon grease into a bowl and mix in cream cheese, Gruyere cheese, butter, and red chili flakes. Refrigerate to set for 15 minutes. Remove and mold into walnut-sized balls. Roll in the crumbled bacon. Plate and serve.

Per serving: Cal 538; Net Carbs 0.5g; Fat 50g; Protein 22g

Savory Pan-Fried Cauliflower with Bacon

Ingredients for 4 servings

1 large head cauliflower, cut into florets

10 oz bacon, chopped

1 garlic clove, minced

Salt and black pepper to taste

2 tbsp parsley, finely chopped

Directions and Total Time: approx. 15 minutes

Pour cauliflower in salted boiling water over medium heat and cook for 5 minutes or until soft; drain and set aside. In a skillet, fry bacon until brown and crispy, 5 minutes. Add cauliflower and garlic and sauté until the cauliflower browns slightly. Season with salt and pepper. Garnish with parsley and serve.

Per serving: Cal 243; Net Carbs 3.9g; Fat 21g; Protein 9g

Green Bean & Mozzarella Roast with Bacon

Ingredients for 4 servings

2 tbsp olive oil

1 tsp onion powder

1 egg, beaten

15 oz fresh green beans

5 tbsp grated mozzarella

4 bacon slices, chopped

Directions and Total Time: approx. 30 minutes

Preheat oven to 350 F. Line a baking sheet with parchment paper. In a bowl, mix olive oil, onion and garlic powders, and egg. Add in green beans and mozzarella cheese and toss to coat. Pour the mixture onto the baking sheet and bake until the green beans brown slightly and cheese melts, 20 minutes. Fry bacon in a skillet until crispy and brown. Remove green beans and divide between serving plates. Top with bacon and serve.

Per serving: Cal 208; Net Carbs 2.6g; Fat 19g; Protein 6g

Salami & Cheddar Skewers

Ingredients for 4 servings

¼ cup olive oil

1 tbsp plain vinegar

2 garlic cloves, minced

1 tsp dried Italian herb blend

4 oz hard salami, cubed

¼ cup pitted Kalamata olives

12 oz cheddar cheese, cubed

1 tsp chopped parsley

Directions and Total Time: approx. 10 min + chilling time

In a bowl, mix olive oil, vinegar, garlic, and herb blend. Add in salami, olives, and cheddar cheese. Mix until well coated. Cover the bowl with plastic wrap and marinate in the refrigerator for 4 hours. Remove, drain the marinade and thread one salami cube, one olive, and one cheese cube on a skewer. Repeat making more skewers with the remaining ingredients. Garnish with the parsley and serve.

Per serving: Cal 585; Net Carbs 1.8g; Fat 52g; Protein 27g

Dessert

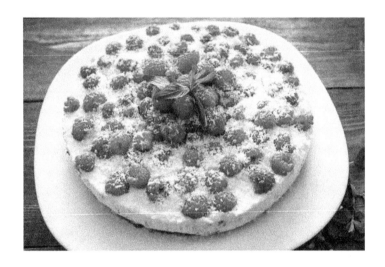

Raspberry Coconut Cheesecake

Ingredients for 6 servings

2 egg whites

1 ¼ cups erythritol

3 cups desiccated coconut

1 tsp coconut oil

¼ cup melted butter

3 tbsp lemon juice

6 ounces raspberries

1 cup whipped cream

3 tbsp lemon juice

24 ounces cream cheese

Directions and Total Time: approx. 40 min + chilling time

Preheat oven to 350 F. Grease a baking pan with coconut oil and line with parchment paper. Mix egg whites, ¼ cup of erythritol, coconut, and butter until a crust forms and pour into the pan. Bake for 25 minutes. Let cool. Beat the cream cheese until soft. Add lemon juice and the remaining erythritol. In another bowl, beat the heavy cream with an electric mixer. Fold the whipped cream into the cheese cream mixture; stir in raspberries. Spread the filling onto the baked crust. Refrigerate for 4 hours. Serve.

Per serving: Cal 215; Net Carbs 3g; Fat 25g; Protein 5g

Peanut Butter & Chocolate Ice Cream Bars

Ingredients for 6 servings

¼ cup cocoa butter pieces, chopped

2 cups heavy whipping cream

⅔ cup peanut butter, softened

1 ½ cups almond milk

1 tbsp vegetable glycerin

6 tbsp xylitol

¾ cup coconut oil

2 oz unsweetened chocolate

Directions and Total Time: approx. 4 hours 20 minutes

Blend heavy cream, peanut butter, almond milk, vegetable glycerin, and half of xylitol until smooth. Place in an ice cream maker and follow the instructions. Spread the ice cream into a lined pan and freeze for 4 hours. Mix coconut oil, cocoa butter, chocolate, and remaining xylitol and microwave until melted; let cool slightly. Slice the ice cream into bars. Dip into the chocolate mixture. Serve.

Per serving: Cal 345 Net Carbs 5 g; Fat 32g; Protein 4g

Lemon-Yogurt Mousse

Ingredients for 4 servings

24 oz plain yogurt, strained overnight in a cheesecloth

2 cups swerve confectioner's sugar

2 lemons, juiced and zested

1 cup whipped cream + extra for garnish

Directions and Total Time: approx. 5 min + cooling time

Whip the plain yogurt in a bowl with a hand mixer until light and fluffy. Mix in the swerve sugar, lemon juice, and salt. Fold in the whipped cream to combine. Spoon the mousse into serving cups and refrigerate for 1 hour. Swirl with extra whipped cream and garnish with lemon zest.

Per serving: Cal 223; Net Carbs 3g; Fat 18g; Protein 12g

Strawberry Chocolate Mousse

Ingredients for 4 servings

1 cup fresh strawberries, sliced

3 eggs

1 cup dark chocolate chips

1 cup heavy cream

1 vanilla extract

1 tbsp swerve sugar

Directions and Total Time: approx. 30 minutes

Melt the chocolate in a microwave-safe bowl in the microwave oven for 1 minute; let cool for 8 minutes. In a bowl, whip the heavy cream until very soft. Whisk in the eggs, vanilla extract, and swerve sugar. Fold in the cooled chocolate. Divide the mousse between glasses, top with the strawberry and chill in the fridge. Serve.

Per serving: Cal 400; Net Carbs 1.7g; Fat 25g; Protein 8g

Maple Lemon Cake

Ingredients for 4 servings

4 eggs

1 cup sour cream

2 lemons, zested and juiced

1 tsp vanilla extract

2 cups almond flour

2 tbsp coconut flour

2 tsp baking powder

½ cup xylitol

1 tsp cardamom powder

½ tsp ground ginger

A pinch of salt

¼ cup maple syrup

Directions and Total Time: approx. 30 minutes

Preheat oven to 400 F. Grease a cake pan with melted butter. In a bowl, beat eggs, sour cream, lemon juice, and vanilla extract until smooth. In another bowl, whisk almond and coconut flours, baking powder, xylitol, cardamom, ginger, salt, lemon zest, and half of maple syrup. Combine both mixtures until smooth and pour the batter into the pan. Bake for 25 minutes or until a toothpick inserted comes out clean. Transfer to a wire rack, let cool, and drizzle with the remaining maple syrup. Serve sliced.

Per serving: Cal 441; Net Carbs 8.5g; Fat 29g; Protein 33g

Saffron & Cardamom Coconut Bars

Ingredients for 4 servings

3 ½ ounces ghee

10 saffron threads

1 ⅓ cups coconut milk

1 ¾ cups shredded coconut

4 tbsp sweetener

1 tsp cardamom powder

Directions and Total Time: approx. 15 min + chilling time

Combine the shredded coconut with 1 cup of coconut milk. In another bowl, mix the remaining coconut milk with the sweetener and saffron. Let sit for 30 minutes, and then combine the two mixtures. Heat the ghee in a wok. Add in the mixture and cook for 5 minutes on low heat, stirring continuously. Mix in cardamom and cook for 5 more minutes. Spread the mixture onto a greased baking pan. Freeze for 2 hours. Cut into bars and serve.

Per serving: Cal 130; Net Carbs 1.4g; Fat 12g; Protein 2g

Granny Smith Apple Tart

Ingredients for 6 servings

2 cups almond flour

¼ cup + 6 tbsp butter

1 ¼ tsp cinnamon

1 cup sweetener

2 cups sliced Granny Smith

½ tsp lemon juice

Directions and Total Time: approx. 45 minutes

Preheat oven to 375 F. Combine 6 tbsp of butter, almond flour, 1 tsp of cinnamon, and ⅓ cup of sweetener in a bowl. Press this mixture into a greased pan. Bake for 5 minutes. Combine apples and lemon juice in a bowl and arrange them on top of the crust. Combine the remaining butter and sweetener and brush over the apples. Bake for 30 minutes. Dust with remaining cinnamon and serve.

Per serving: Cal 302; Net Carbs 6.7g; Fat 26g; Protein 7g

Chocolate Mocha Ice Bombs

Ingredients for 4 servings

½ pound cream cheese

4 tbsp powdered sweetener

2 ounces strong coffee

2 tbsp cocoa powder

1 ounce cocoa butter, melted

2 ½ oz dark chocolate, melted

Directions and Total Time: approx. 10 min + chilling time

Combine cream cheese, sweetener, coffee, and cocoa powder in a food processor. Roll 2 tbsp of the mixture and place on a lined tray. Mix the melted cocoa butter and chocolate and coat the bombs with it. Freeze for 2 hours.

Per serving: Cal 127; Net Carbs 1.4g; Fat 13g; Protein 2g

CPSIA information can be obtained
at www.ICGtesting.com
Printed in the USA
BVHW041206010321
601386BV00008B/643